" *History is not just stone, notable people, and bricks. It includes the reaction of those who were there and the community's ongoing response.*"

—Jim Boles

Vanishing Past Series

This book is part of the Vanishing Past Series published by Vanishing Past Press LLC. Vanishing Past Press is dedicated to the documentation, preservation, and distribution of works of scholarship and cultural importance with emphasis on under-examined or unexplored topics. This book is part of that effort.

Publisher: Vanishing Past Press
Designer: Rachel Bridges
Technical Advisor: Michelle Green

Top cover image: This is a Schnee Four Cell Bath. This would
have been used by the healing baths and water cure doctors. It
promised relief for joint pain and rheumatic conditions and to
stimulate blood circulation. It was popular in these alternative
medicine facilities because the patient did not have to undress,
and a continuous water supply was not needed.

Bottom cover image: Dr Schmith's Sanitarium,
471 Market street, Lockport, New York

ISBN: 978-1-949860-00-9

NO HARM WAS DONE

Alternative Medicine in Lockport, New York 1830- 1930

James M. Boles

Editor's Note: The exact language of this time has been retained for historical accuracy. No offense is intended toward any individual or group.

Dedication

To all those who contribute to local history:
citizens, students, researchers, librarians,
booksellers and historians.

James M. Boles, EdD

Table of Contents

Introduction

*N*o Harm Was Done—Alternative Medicine in Lockport, New York, is based upon a series of researched articles published in the *Lockport Union Sun and Journal* in 2016 and 2017.

I have been studying health and healing in the Western New York area for many years. When researching the book *When There Were Poorhouses*, I came across a number of commercial businesses that were based upon an alternative view of health and healing that differed from the traditional (often called allopathic) medicine of the time. The mainstream medicine practiced in the 1800s into the early 1900s was primitive. Doctors often were untrained and science lacking, and licensing was not formalized. Bleeding, ingestion of poisonous mercury and other toxic substances, and surgeries were heavily used, and people had little confidence in traditional doctors.

The alternative medical providers, who were local Western New York healers, used a variety of vibrant aids to help their patients. Allopathic (traditional) medicine at the time could be much more dangerous.

CHAPTER 1
The Healers

Dr. B.W. Dean "The Sweat Doctor" Thompsonian Botanic System Practitioner Lockport, New York, 1841

Benjamin W. Dean was born in 1794 at Philipsburg Manor, Westchester County, New York. For his medical training, Dr. Dean studied under a traditional physician. In 1825, he is listed as the physician for Macedon Center, New York, a canal town just east of Rochester. In 1841, Dr. Dean, his wife, Sophia, and son, Herman were living in Lockport, New York, where he practiced "sweat doctor" medicine.

The new method Dr. Dean was using in Lockport was invented by Dr. Thompson of Ohio. It was a system and book that sold for $20.00 and included a stock of available medicines that could be purchased by the practitioner and recipes to make homemade cures; extracts from Native American vegetables were favored. This was a nontraditional medicine that was advertised as an alternative to the medicine practiced at the time. Dr. Thompson, the inventor of the system, believed that disease was caused by a clogged system. This would be helped by purging and sweating. Doctors who used this method were sometimes called "Sweat Doctors."

REFORMED
MEDICAL PRACTICE.

DR. B. W. DEAN

For 20 years a practitioner in the old school of medicine and surgery, of the State of New York, has, for good reasons, abandoned the popular method of treating diseases by blood-letting, calomel, and all poisonous minerals and drugs, and has for two years past adopted the

THOMPSONIAN BOTANIC SYSTEM OF PRACTICE.

If the friends of this system in the vicinity of

LOCKPORT

wish to patronize a practice of experience in both systems they can do so by calling on Doct. Dean at his

☞ *Office over the Drug Store two doors west* 🖑

☞ *of the Canal Bank* 🖑

P.S.   All kinds of Thompsonian

BOTANIC MEDICINES

on hand for sale, as low as can be purchased elsewhere.

Lockport, March 25, 1841

Printed at the Niagara Courier Office – Lockport, NY

Local flyer from Dr. Dean with an announcement of the Thompsonian Botanic Medicine System.

Shortly after publishing this flyer, Dr. Dean passed away on September 10, 1841, at the age of forty-seven. Dr. Benjamin W. Dean is buried at Cold Springs Cemetery in the Town of Lockport in the Price family section. Dr. Dean's sister married into the Price family.

I want to thank the officials at the Cold Springs Cemetery, Lockport, New York, for their assistance in locating the grave.

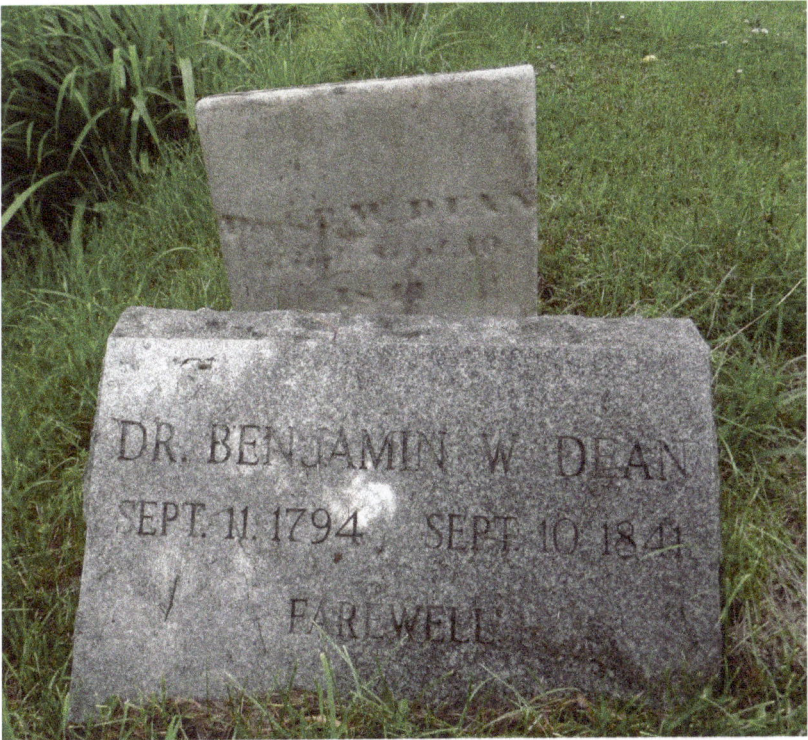

J. Boles 2015

Dr. Dean has two headstones. The worn original stone was replaced by a new stone, but the original one remains. Cold Springs Cemetery, Lockport, New York

H. Knapp, MD, Water-Cure Physician, 1851–1855 Lockport, New York

Dr. Knapp was a practitioner of alternative medicine. He was also a lecturer on the new medicine of hydropathy and the evils of the "old school medicine." Dr. Knapp was based in Niagara County, New York, with an office at the corner of Church and Grand Streets. In another listing in 1854, he had an office over Days Variety Store where he was promoted as a Water-Cure physician and surgeon. In 1853, he proposed to start a Water-Cure in Niagara Falls, but there is no record that the facility opened. Dr. Knapp, a frequent contributor, was often mentioned in *The Water-Cure Journal.*

Hydropathy was a therapy that used water to treat a disease or condition. Hot, tepid, and cold mineral water was often used in baths and/or under pressure as part of the treatments. Versions of hydropathy are still used today.

Water-Cure Therapy had wide-ranging claims for its benefits. Cures for pains, insomnia, mental disorders, addictions, and arthritis were frequently mentioned.

... Old fogies and drug doctors will receive no money at my hands. I expect to start a Water-Cure at Niagara Falls in the Spring. Thus you see I am unsettled just now. When I get the apparatus you shall hear from me again.

Respectfully,
H. Knapp, M.D.

The Water-Cure Journal, *Vol. 15, No 1. An early publication that focused on products, physics, facilities, and Water-Cure treatments. Published by Joel Shaw, MD, Editor, 56 Bond Street, New York, New York.*

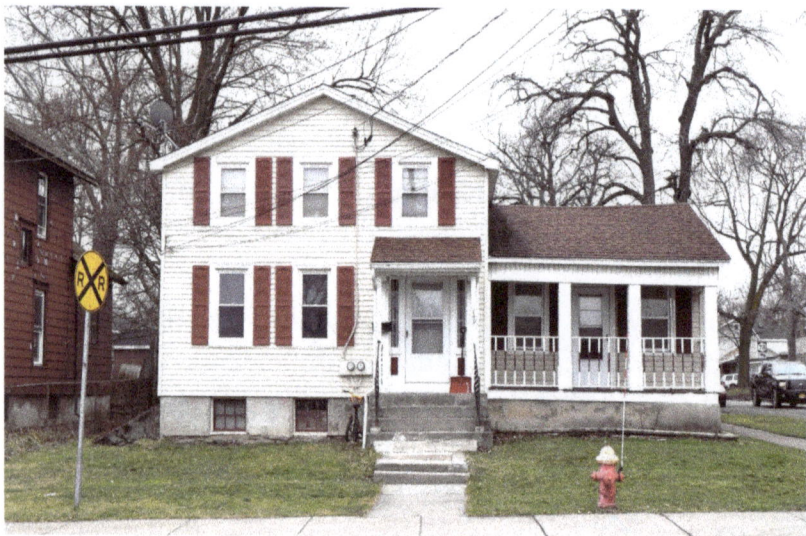

J. Boles 2016

In the 1850s, Dr. H. Knapp's office was located on the south-west corner of Church and Grand Streets, Lockport, New York.

Lecturers: The subscriber having purchased the most splendid and extensive lecturing apparatus in the world, comprising the best French Manikins, Skeletons, (models) of all parts of the (human) system, and extensive specimens of Morbid Anatomy of all kind of diseases with over fifteen hundred superior paintings and drawings, brilliantly illustrating in life-like colors every part of the system and characters of life, all of which have recently been transported from Paris, is prepared, from a long experience in public lecturing, to give courses of scientific, useful, and amusing lectures on the laws of Health and Philosophy of Life. Literary societies and others wishing for his services, will be attended to by addressing him at Lockport, Niagara Co., N.Y.

H. Knapp, M.D.

The Water-Cure Journal, *Vol. 17, October 20, 1855.*

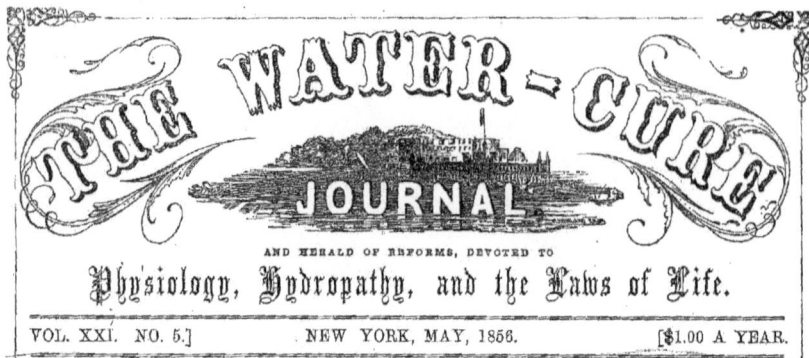

Heading for The Water-Cure Journal – *May 1856.*

Dr. Knapp was a prolific writer on the treatment of diseases by the Water-Cure. Here is a quote from one of his long articles on the subject.

> "Eight years' experience in Hydropathy has suggested to me many changes in the use of water, that I have found improvements on the early methods of using it. The first change I would mention, and which I deem the most important, is the use of *tepid* instead of *cold* water. I am certain that injury has been done, not only to individuals, but to the Water-Cure system, by the too free use of cold water."

After 1855, Dr. Knapp's Water-Cure practice was not found in any Lockport, New York, directories.

Thank you to the Niagara County Historian's Office for assistance with this research.

Dr. T. Teasdill
Lockport's Blind Charm Doctor

Dr. John T. Teasdill was born in 1794 in England and shows up in ads starting in 1853 in the *Lockport Daily Courier* and the *Lockport Directory* (1859), where he was listed as a physician with a house at 39 Vine Street. In 1868, he moved his home and office to 2 Vine Street.

---

12   LOCKPORT CITY DIRECTORY

Dr. John T. Teasdill,
No. 2 Vine St., East Lockport, N.Y.,

Undertakes the cure of diseases, with or without medicine, or by simply laying hands on the patient, when all other means have failed. Dr. Teasdill has effected wonderful and thorough cures. He has succeeded in bringing away Reptiles and other animals from the Stomach.

Patients at a distance can have information of their disease by simply sending the Doctor their symptoms, name and age, enclosing 3 cent stamp.

HE ALSO CURES CANCERS BY THE SAME PROCESS.

His professional ads list some unusual results with success "in bringing away Reptiles and other animals from the Stomach." Lockport City Directory 1871— Dr. John T. Teasdill.

While in Lockport in his seventies, it is rumored that Teasdill married a young girl who left him, stealing his money. Shortly after this incident, Dr. Teasdill moved to Buffalo, New York, and practiced a short time at the Buehl-owned building on Franklin Street, before he died at seventy-nine years of age in 1873. Dr. Teasdill's early story can only be found in a few ads in local papers and directories. Likely because of his surprising practices, his death was covered extensively by the local papers and later by Niagara County Historian Clarence O. Lewis.

The Doctor seemed to die a natural death, but the curious objects found in his office made for sensational reading. Clarence O. Lewis mentions in his April 1, 1959, article that "Flasks of quick silver, a prayer book containing six squirrel tails, and incantations against the powers of darkness and evil, written in blood." A charm was found around his neck that contained a horseshoe, a stuffed frog, a Hazelnut, and an English silver shilling piece.

Despite the divergent care he offered, it looks like Teasdill had a thriving practice in both Lockport and Buffalo. Why did he come to Lockport, New York? Where did he receive his training? Where was he buried? Was he a witch doctor? All of this is unknown. He is a wildly interesting character from Lockport's past.

Thank you to the Niagara County Historian's Office and the Lockport Public Library for help with this research.

Doctor Schmith's Medical Dispensary and Sanitarium Lockport, New York

Dr. W.J. Schmith, a homeopathic physician, set up his first practice in 1900 at 118 John Street, Lockport, New York. It is believed that Dr. Schmith moved to Lockport from Martinsville in Niagara County where he was listed in the *Medical Society of New York Directory*, Volume 12, 1882.

In 1901, Dr. W.J. Schmith moved to a larger facility at 471 Market Street, overlooking the canal, and opened the Schmith Medical Dispensary and Sanitarium (1901–1908). This large stone house was built in 1829 by Edward Bissel and was later the home of Lyman Spalding.

Sanitariums were known for convalescent care. It is believed Schmith had live-in facilities for his longer-term patients. Dr. Schmith's listings in local directories mentioned that he was an Herb Doctor.

Homeopathic Medicine

This is an alternative system of treatments that uses very small doses of minerals, plants, and other extracts to assist the body in its healing process. Samuel Hahnemann, MD, is credited with the founding of homeopathy. His healing theory was "that which can produce a set of symptoms in a healthy individual, can treat a sick individual who is manifesting a similar set of symptoms." For example, the plant Hypericum, also known as St. John's Wort, is used for diseases of the nervous system.

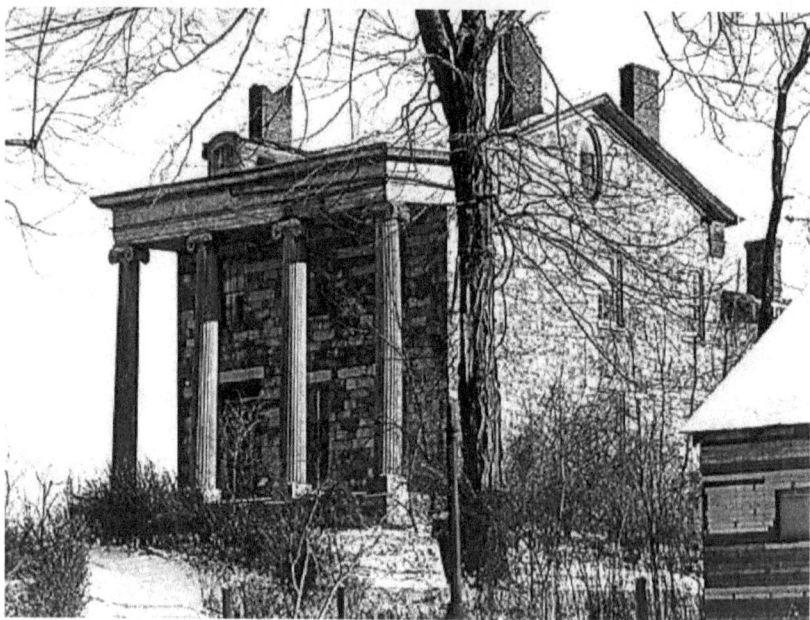

471 Market Street, Lockport, New York. Photo 1946.

Research indicates that Dr. Schmith sold his sanitarium and moved his practice to Buffalo, New York, in 1908.

"$10,000 worth of property for sale for $4,500; 23 years to pay it in and no interest to pay. $1,200 down, balance payable $12 per month. Take large stone house, a perfect mansion in good condition. Barn and other out houses, three acres of land. Plenty of fruit, good water. Must be seen to be appreciated. 471 Market Street. Lockport, NY

Dr. W.J. Schmith."

Binghamton Press, December 1907.

Plate 2

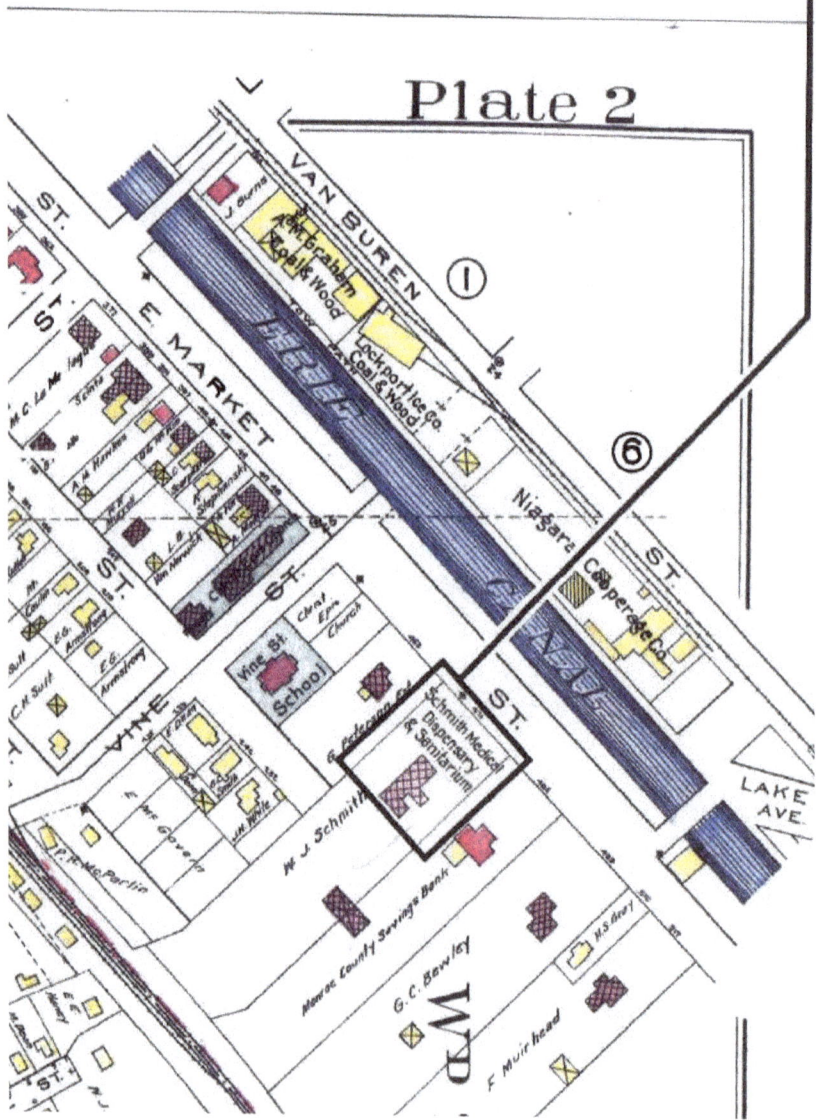

Town of Lockport Map, 1908.

What's There Now?

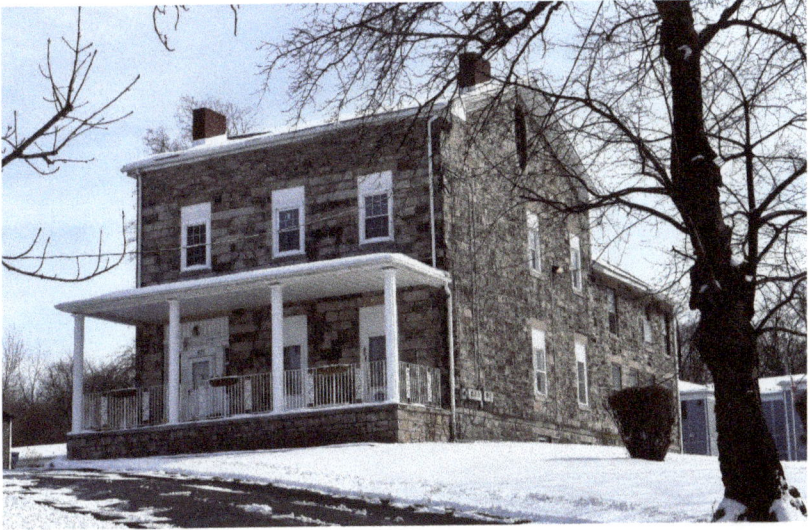

J. Boles 2019

471 Market Street—Home of Schmith Medical Dispensary and Sanitarium.

Professor Wamon

Professor Wamon, the "Magnetic Healer," was based at the Magnetic Institute, located at 74 Walnut Street, Lockport, New York, in the 1800s. He traveled to local towns, including Wilson, Somerset, Lyndonville, and Medina offering magnetic healing to those in need. An ad in the *Lockport Journal* in 1889, titled "Professor Wamon's Public Healing!" listed his many skills. The report also mentioned:

> "He is certainly endowed with an astonishing and phenomenal healing gift, and these bold, public exhibitions of his beneficent power, have now placed its absolute genuineness and the reality of his singular cures beyond all doubt. The cures witnessed and carefully investigated by our reporter, he asserts, exceed in marvelousness any of the apparently incredible testimonials that have been so often advertised in the Journal in the past."

Further on in the article/advertisement, there are many stories of his miracle cures in local towns. Here is an example from Newfane, New York:

"Mrs. Hern lay on a sofa and had long been unable to walk from inflammatory rheumatism. Within five seconds, she started up, ran and leaped several times, and next day amazed everybody by walking to church."

The belief was that as the professor placed his hands on the patient, magnetic radiation energy was passed from his powerful hands through the patient's body, assisting in the healing process.

Magnetic healing was promoted as a drug-free approach to curing illness. The drugs that were available and utilized by the traditional physicians at the time could be dangerous to your health.

Professor Wamon was practicing his healing skills at a time when colleges, the government, and the American Medical Association (AMA) were trying to standardize and license doctors, as there were many paths to becoming a doctor, and many medical schools, some of questionable quality. The professor, who never claimed to be a physician, avoided this scrutiny.

Doctor Daniel Lester

According to city directories, Dr. Daniel Lester practiced in the Lockport area from the 1880s onward, with his first Electro-Medicated Bath at 144 Washburn Street. Eventually, in 1887, his facility, now named the Electro Therapeutic Bath, moved to 131 Church Street at Green Street. This large sandstone building is listed in the *Index of Stone Buildings*, which indicates that the house was once the residence of Patrick J. Hopkins, a blacksmith, with S. Parmele and Dr. Lester also named as past owners. *The Index of Stone Buildings*, compiled by Teresa Lasher, can be found at the Niagara County Historians Office.

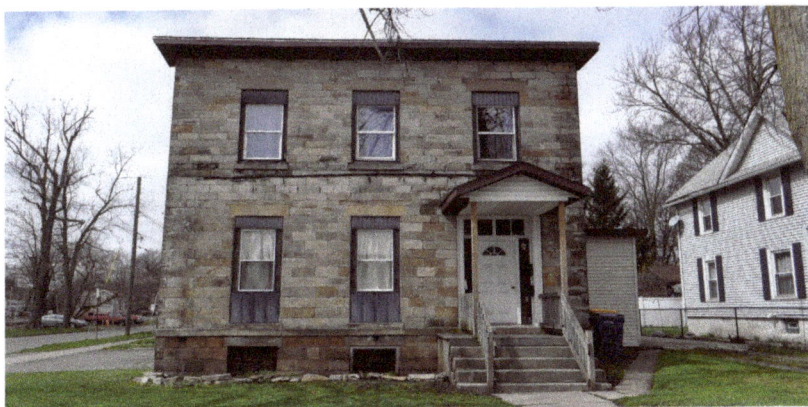

J. Boles 2017

Dr. Lester's Electro Therapeutic Baths, 131 Church Street at the corner of Green Street, Lockport, New York

Dr. Lester was educated at the Virginia Eclectic Medical College, which was located in Philadelphia. As an Eclectic Physician, Dr. Lester would have been trained in the use of nontraditional medicine. Eclectic physicians considered themselves open to a plan of treatment that would fit the patient; they were educated in the use of herbal medicines and alternative practices, which contrasted with the mainstream (traditional) allopathic medicine of the time.

Dr. Lester also offered Electro-Therapeutic Baths as a treatment. These baths could range from an early tanning bed to a machine producing low-level electric current through sponges placed on the body. They could also involve the use of hot and cold water and vapor.

Eclectic medicine was a reaction against the established medical treatments of the era. There were many Eclectic Medical Schools; some were legitimate with a prescribed course of study, and others have been now labeled diploma mills. The last Eclectic Medical School closed in 1939. Before medical education was research-based, with schools certified and physicians licensed, much of the education was of unquantifiable quality.

As traditional medicine struggled with a questionable reputation, there developed a market for alternative healers. In early Lockport, there was Rattlesnake John who sold boiled down snake fat as a cure for rheumatism and other ailments. Doctor Dean the "Sweat Doctor" and Dr. Knapp, who practiced hydrotherapy and operated a Water Cure just up the street from Dr. Lester's Electro Therapeutic Baths. Sleights Mineral Baths was a few blocks away, as well as Dr. Teasdill the "Charm Doctor," and many others who operated in the city as well.

In 1905, Dr. Lester and his wife, Mary, are listed in the city directory as living at 186 Green Street, Lockport, New York, not far down the street from his Electro-Therapeutic Baths.

CHAPTER 2
Alternative Health Products

Rattlesnake John, Snake Oil Vendor, Lockport, New York

When Lockport was first settled by white settlers, it was very primitive, unspoiled, heavily wooded, and swampy. In the August 11, 1873, *Lockport Daily Courier*, Edna Deane Smith is interviewed in a series of articles titled "Recollections of an Early Settler." Here she mentions the rattlesnakes.

> "The rocky borders and sides of the ravine or basin, in which the Locks are, were filled with fissures and scams, in which they congregated. The Northern bank was the favorite home of the reptiles. The rocks were bare of earth and the fissures in the rocks were many of them not more than five or six inches in width, and twenty or thirty in depth. In the Spring they would come out to sun themselves, and parties of the more adventurous would go out to kill them. Everyone considered it a duty to dispose of as many of these reptiles as possible, and a young man would return from a ramble in the woods dragging a dead rattlesnake behind him…"

A popular phrase for peddler of fraudulent medicine is "Snake Oil Salesman," but in the early nineteenth century, Lockport had a genuine Snake Oil Salesman who sold a real Snake Oil boiled from the rattlesnakes found in Lockport.

This man, called locally "Rattlesnake John," did his hunting along the Lockport hillsides. The road that cut through his hunting area is still known as Rattlesnake Hill. So strong was the image of the rattlesnakes and the escarpment that in the 1830s, William Wallace Whitmore opened a quarry near Rattlesnake Hill and promptly branded his Medina Sandstone as "Rattlesnake Stone."

Although Rattlesnake John moved on to "Beyond Lake Michigan" when the supply of snakes diminished, there was still a news item in the *Lockport Daily Journal* on June 7, 1879, which mentioned Rattlesnake Oil as a medicine for the cure of rheumatism.

Late News Items.

- Rattlesnake oil sells in New York for $1 an ounce. It is said to be an excellent ointment for the cure of rheumatism.

Thank you to the Lockport Public Library for their assistance.

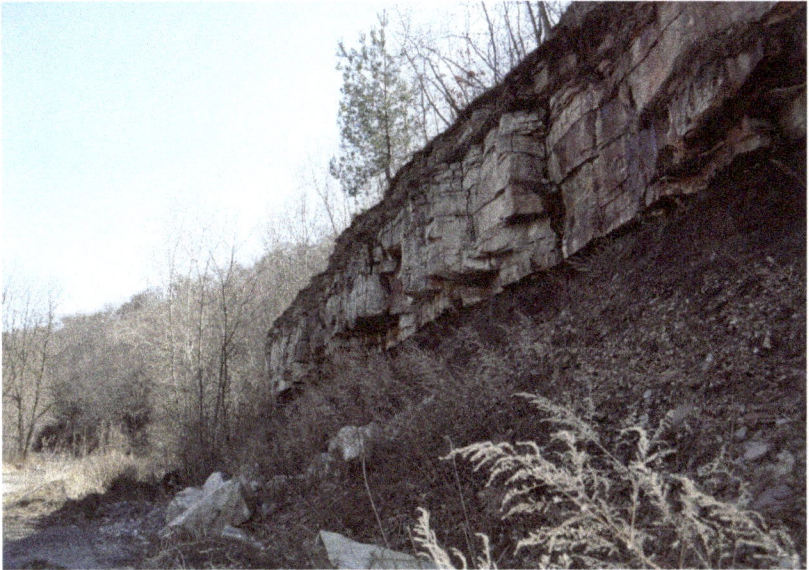

The Lockport Escarpment on Rattlesnake Hill, John's hunting area.

Lockport's Early Health Food
Franklin Mills Wheat Flour
and Wheatlet
731 Garden Street, Lockport, New York

T he south bank of the canal beside the locks was home to many factories that utilized the powerful mill races to produce their products.

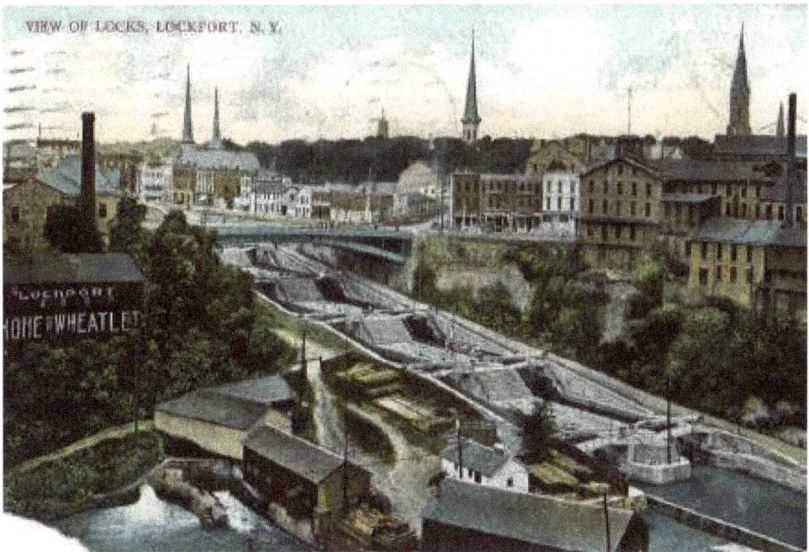

Franklin Mills Wheatlet advertising on the Old Spaulding Mills Storage Building.

With a large painted Wheatlet sign on the side of a building, the Franklin Mills Company stood out to those traveling on the canal. It is also visible on the many period postcards of the locks at Lockport, New York. The business address of the company was 731 Spring Street, corner of Garden Street.

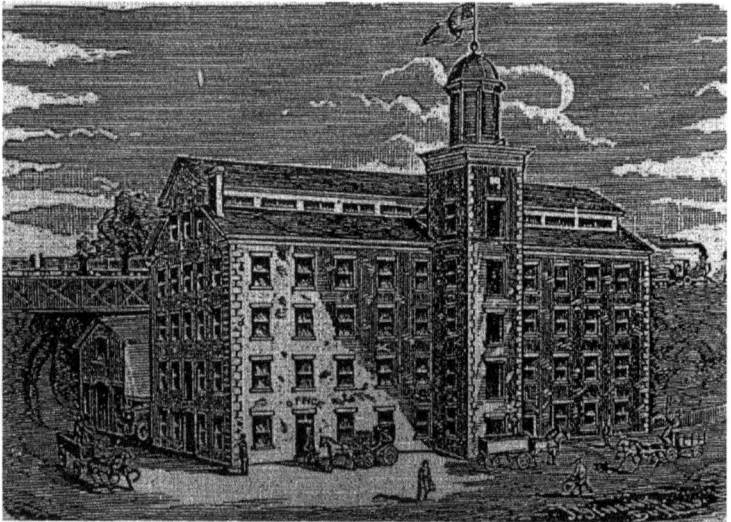

731 Spring Street. Franklin Mill Company, Lockport, New York. There were six floors in the factory. Lockport Public Library History Room— Binder Lockport Industries.

This is a distance from the canal and the mill race that was on the south bank. How did the mill receive waterpower? I reached out to an expert on the canal mill races, Dr. Scott Geise. From Geise's records, the Franklin Mills factory received power from both the south mill race and 18 Mile Creek. At the time of the mills operation the mill race left the canal bank and ran southeast crossing under Market Street and continued to Garden Street and the Franklin Mills factory on Garden Street. This research indicates that the remains of the 1833 building can now be found at 31 Exchange Street.

The Franklin Mills Company had many health declarations for their main products, Wheatlet—a breakfast food, and the Franklin Mills Flour.

THE FRANKLIN MILLS COMPANY

The fine flour of the entire wheat, ground by the Franklin Mills Company, Lockport, N.Y., containing as it does all the phosphates, mineral salts, and gluten of the entire wheat, is recommended by many physicians for use in the preparation of food for those suffering from weak stomach, because it is easily digestible. Nourishing as it does every part of the body, it is held to be especially valuable in the diet of children.

Attention is directed to the advertisement of the Franklin Mills Company on another page of this issue.

American Medico-Surgical Bulletin, 1897.

Wheatlet was described as an unrefined/unbleached natural food with promises for relief of nervousness, indigestion, irritability, a morose disposition (sullen), and help with "clever" work, such as writing.

Franklin Wheat Flour claimed to be "The fine flower of the entire wheat" and a brain food. It would help every nerve tissue and feed the nerves. The nervous and debilitated would be assisted.

The Franklin Mills building dates back to 1833 and was once owned by the Governor Washington Hunt family. The Franklin Mills Company occupied the building from 1877 to 1907 when the structure was destroyed in a November 4 fire. After the fire, the company was reorganized and consolidated their operations to Batavia, New York.

Thank you to the Niagara County Historical Society, Niagara County Historians Office, the Lockport Public Library, Dr. Scott Geise, and realtor Maureen Walck.

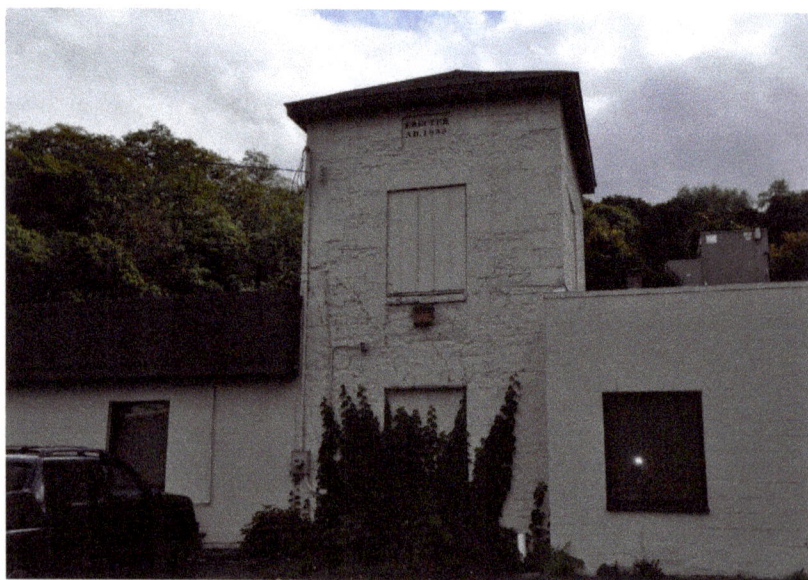

Today what remains of the Franklin Mills building can be found at 31 Exchange Street. The center stone section has a stone block at the top dated 1833.

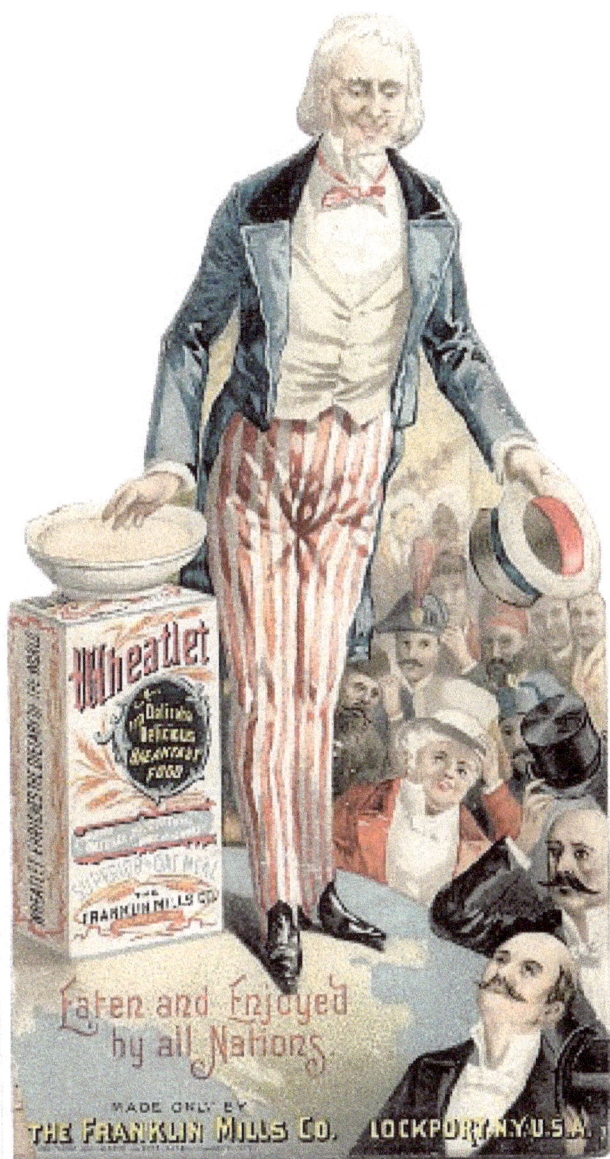

The US government Commissary Department was a customer of the Franklin Mill Co., and their ads highlight this endorsement.

Uncle Charlie Perry
Lockport's Spokesperson for
Duffy's Pure Malt Whiskey—A Medicine

Although a Rochester, New York, product, Duffy's Pure Malt Whiskey had a Lockport connection with a ninety-two-year-old Lockport resident as its main spokesperson promoting the healthy virtues of the distilled beverage. In the ads, "Uncle Charlie" claimed that Duffy's kept him young and proposed vigorous and constant use of the drink. He felt that it built nerve tissues preventing decay and kept the system in a normal healthy condition. Samuel Charles Perry was born in New York State and worked as a farmer. With a regular dose of Duffy's Malt Whiskey, "Uncle Charlie" Perry lived until the age of ninety-five. He died in 1912 after a brief illness lasting four days. The average life expectancy in 1912 for a male was fifty-one years. Did Duffy's Pure Malt Whiskey give Uncle Charlie that extra forty-four years?

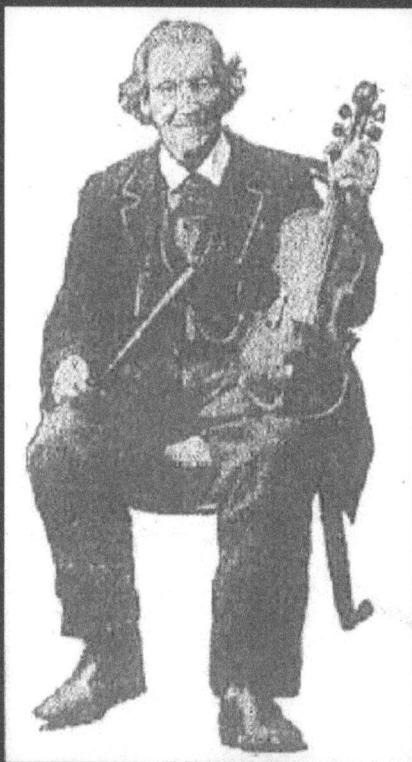

1909 ad featuring Lockport resident, Uncle Charlie Perry

"Uncle Charlie" Perry 92 Years Young

Mr. Samuel Charles Perry, of Lockport, N.Y. who is 92 years old and a bachelor, retains all his faculties to a remarkable degree.

"In my extreme old age I am exercising the same discretion with but the one exception that I find Duffy's Pure Malt Whiskey an indispensable medicine. As a tonic and general preserver of health in old age I believe that it has no equal."

Duffy's Pure Malt Whiskey is a predigested food which has a stimulating and tonic effect upon the system.

Duffy's Malt Whiskey, a new product in 1886, had medical claims that helped buffer the ongoing threats of the Temperance Movement. It was sold in both bars and drugstores, as malt products were considered to be medicinal. Duffy's Malt Whiskey had declarations as a remedy for pneumonia, nervous prostration, insomnia, loss of mental powers, and female weaknesses. The company closed in 1926 with the pressures of Prohibition.

In the 1910 Federal census, Town of Lockport, New York, a Charles Perry, ninety-three years of age, is listed as living with relatives, the Prentice family on Turnpike Road, Route 104, and is recorded as related to Herbert A. Prentice as an uncle. Just up the road is a new business that makes several varieties of whiskey Uncle Charlie might have enjoyed. Opened in 2015 at 4408 Ridge Road, Lockport, is Niagara Craft Spirits Distillery. I talked with Todd Snyder, a whiskey expert, about malt whiskey. Todd said, "Whiskey is regulated by the Department of Treasury's Alcohol and Tobacco Tax and Trade Bureau (TTB). By their definition, Malt Whiskey is made from a mash of at least 51% barley malt which is fermented and then distilled at 160 Proof or less. After distillation, the spirit is then aged in charred new oak containers at 125 Proof or less." He then mentioned that they plan to produce a malt whiskey similar to the malt whiskey from Uncle Charlie's time. I suggested they consider Uncle Charlie's legacy when they name the product.

Thank you to the Niagara County Historical Society, the Niagara County Historians Office, Deputy Clerk Judi Newbold of the Town of Lockport Clerks Office, and Todd Snyder at Niagara Craft Spirits Distillery.

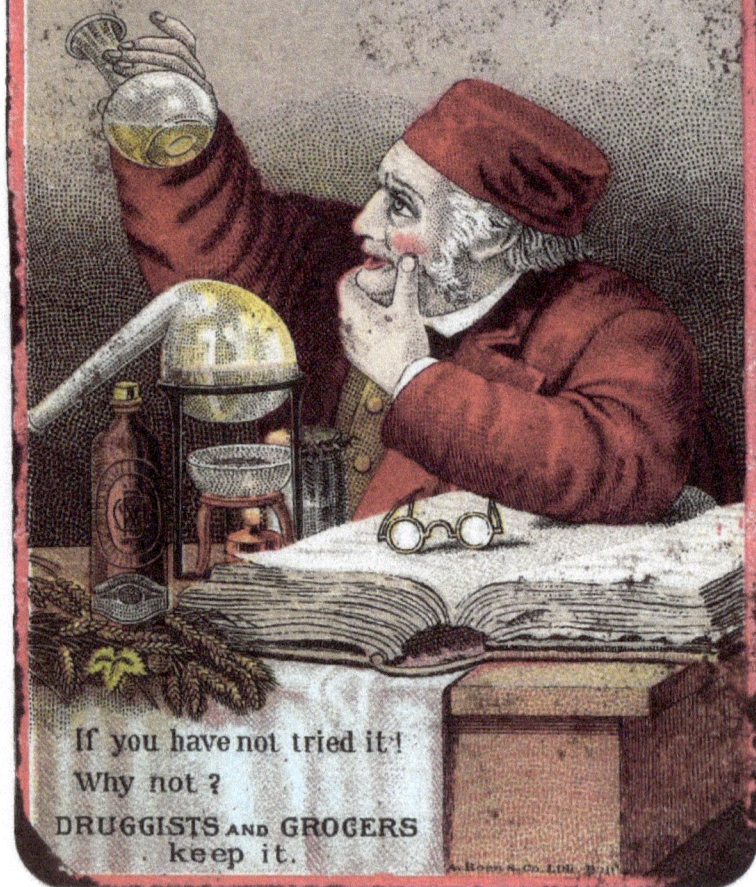

Early ad for Duffy's Malt Whiskey.

CHAPTER 3
Healing Facilities

The Health Baths of Main Street, Part One

Before there was a bath in every home, there were a series of earlier cleansing baths along Main Street in Lockport. Used by local residents and canal travelers, the baths offered by Lyman Spalding on the south canal bank and the fancy shaving saloon at Main and Pine Streets, operated by Fred Specht, are two well-known examples of these cleansing baths. Specht added hot and cold baths in 1872; however, neither of these baths had health claims.

HOME 674   BELL 407-J

MRS. M. L. EVANS

Steam Baths, Massages and Electric Treatments

ADELLA A. EVANS

Hair Dressing,   Facial and Scalp Treatments,
        Shampooing,   Weaving, Manicuring
Over 6 Main Street   Lockport, N. Y.

1911 Lockport Directory.

The health baths, in contrast, promoted their alternative therapies and used water and devices to promise cures and well-being. The earliest health bath (in 1910) was located above 6 Main Street. This bath offered Turkish baths and massages operated by Mrs. M.L. Evans.

The Sulphur Vapor Baths 1920–1927

One of the most long-lived of the baths was the facility at 81 Main Street, with the earliest ad appearing in the 1920s. K.L. O'Connell, a nurse, was the operator. This healing business used Sulphur Vapor Baths with the Kruse System.

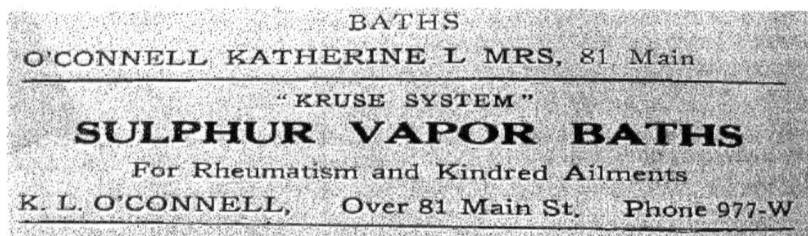

BATHS
O'CONNELL KATHERINE L MRS, 81 Main
"KRUSE SYSTEM"
SULPHUR VAPOR BATHS
For Rheumatism and Kindred Ailments
K. L. O'CONNELL,   Over 81 Main St.   Phone 977-W

1920 Lockport Directory.

The Kruse System, invented by John F. Kruse of Indianapolis, Indiana, was sold mainly in the mid-west and eastern United States. The patient would sit in a cabinet with their head exposed to cold air. Sulphur vapor of various temperatures would be injected into the cabinet. Afterwards, there was a massage.

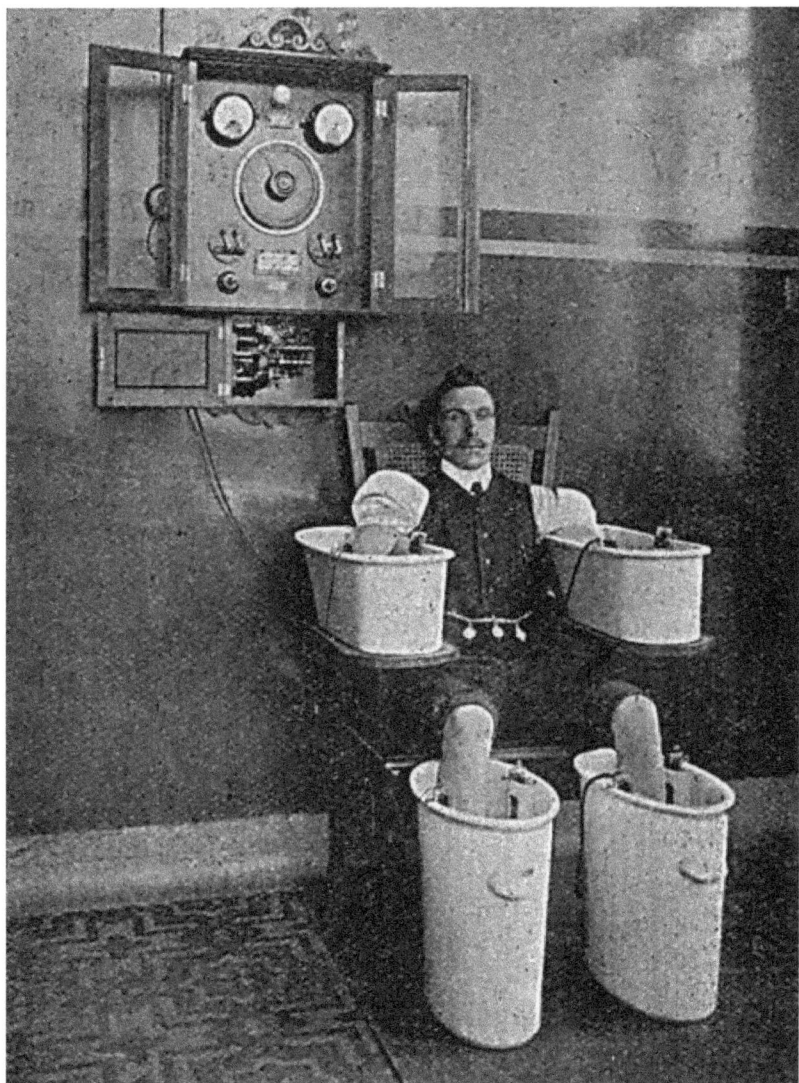

Early Electric Bath; this model is called the Schnee Bath.

Types of Treatments

Sulphur Vapor Baths
Used for pain, skin diseases, liver spots, parasite diseases, and colds.

Electric Baths
Used low levels of current in the water.

Turkish Baths
Hot dry air then a cooling off with cool air or cool water and a massage.

In the next column, we will look at Main Street's most successful bath, The Lockport Health Bath. Thank you to the Lockport Public Library and the Niagara County Historian's Office for their assistance with this research.

The Health Baths of Main Street, Part Two

In this space earlier I covered the cleansing baths of Lyman Spalding and Fred Specht who offered their facilities to the public before there were baths in the home. In 1910, Mrs. M.L. Evans, with the first health bath, offered steam baths, massage, and electric treatments. Today we will look at Lockport's most successful health bath, which operated for over thirty-eight years in the same location.

The Lockport Baths at 81 Main Street 1928–1966

In 1928, the first ad for the new Lockport Baths appears in the *Lockport Directory* with Robert A. Ruth, who was a licensed

14   BATHS

THE LOCKPORT BATHS

(Formerly THE LOCKPORT SULPHUR BATHS)

SULPHUR VAPOR BATHS

ELECTRIC CABINET, MINERAL AND VIT-O-NET BLANKET BATHS.—MASSAGE,—ULTRA VIOLET SUN.—VIBRATORY RE-DUCING TREATMENTS.

ROBERT A. RUTH, Proprietor.   :   Licensed Physio-Therapist

MISS E. M. VENHERM, Assistant

81 MAIN STREET   'PHONE 2157-W   LOCKPORT, N. Y.

1920 Lockport Directory.

physio-therapist (an early name for a physical therapist), listed as the proprietor and Miss E.M. Venherm as his assistant.

Other ads from the late 1920s list Robert A. Ruth as a naturopath, which generally indicates he used natural means of healing. The new baths added a large number of treatments.

Types of Treatments

Sulphur Vapor Baths
Used for pain, skin diseases, liver spots, parasite diseases, and colds.

Electric Cabinet
Used ultraviolet "sunlight" (early tanning booth).

Electric Baths
Used low levels of current in the water.

Mineral Baths
Rids the body of toxins and impurities. The bath uses hot, warm, or cold water. Relieves aches, pains, stress, and nervous concerns.

Blanket Baths
Hot or cold blanket wraps. Rids the body of toxins and impurities, skin diseases, and stress. Can be electric like the Vit-O-Net Blanket.

The business, with Robert Ruth as the owner, operated from 1928 to 1966 when likely it moved because of threatening urban renewal on Main Street and a declining interest in health baths. Robert Ruth moved to the nearby Bewley building, suite 307. From 1966 to 1975, Robert Ruth had his office at the Bewley Building where he was listed as a physio-therapist and then a physical therapist. He retired in 1975, selling his equipment to local practitioners.

Thank you to the Lockport Public Library, the Niagara County Historians Office, and Lockport resident Ruth Ruberto for their assistance with this research.

I have received a question about the early water supply for these facilities. Given their location on the canal and the proximity to the Spalding Mineral Spring on the south canal bank, there was ample water. They used filtered canal water, the Spalding Mineral Spring, which had a large collecting basin behind the buildings on the north side of Main Street, and cistern water. In the early 1900s, the municipal water system was available on Main Street in Lockport.

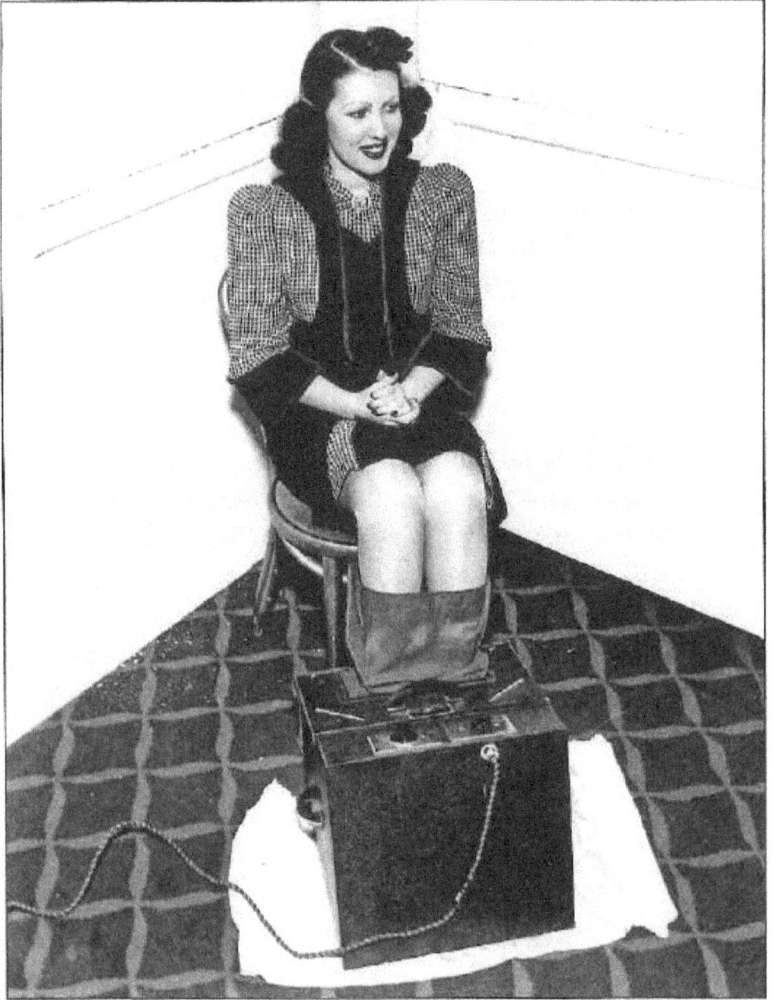

Electric Medicated Vapor Bath, designed to relieve tired muscles, stimulate circulation, and reduce inflammation, is one of the bath treatments

For Physicians
Surgeons and Hospitals

The Vit-O-Net Electrical Blanket system is
proving of inestimable value to members
of the pro-fession desiring an appliance
that stimulates circulation and eliminates
impurities through the pores. It Contains
15,000 feet of protected refined magnet wire
woven into fabric.

Vit-O-Net Mfg. Co.
4111 Ravenswood Ave. Chicago, Ill.

The Vit-O-Net Electrical Blanket System was one of the treatments offered at the Lockport Baths.

The Search for Lockport, New York's Healing Spring at St. Joseph's Academy—Help Needed

O ne of the purposes of this local history column is to have readers help in the search for more information and clues to the many mysteries in the Lockport area. Today's column is part of that search, and I encourage readers to contact me if they have any further knowledge or questions.

In the 1820s, at the time of the opening of the Erie Canal, Joel McCollum bought a large tract of land, over 300 acres, that extended from beyond North Adam Street and bordered on Old Niagara Road to the Erie Canal. The area was not highly settled, and it was undeveloped land.

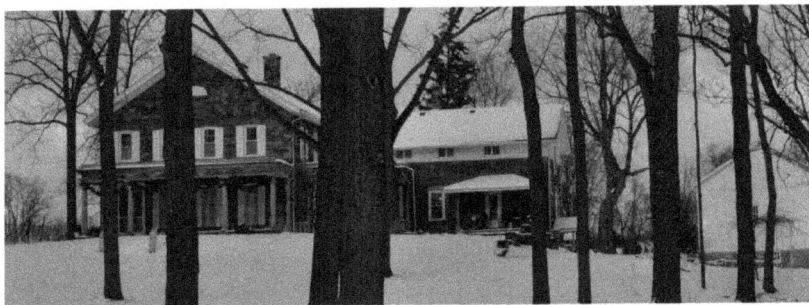

J. Boles 2016

McCollum Farm 254 North Adam Street

In 1877, a particle of the land, with a house and out buildings on both sides of Olcott Street, was transferred to the Sisters of St. Mary of Namur. This order, first established in Belgium, was sent to Lockport to establish Catholic Schools for the many new immigrants. The Sisters' lower town land was named St. Joseph's Academy. It functioned as a school (1889–1891) and a retreat and healing facility for the sick and for members of the order who needed rest (1877–1927). The land was also used for farming. A 1908 map shows the property as St. Joseph's Academy. Some of the property was later sold, and by 1908, the property that remained was a triangle-shaped lot on Olcott Street (Map 1908).

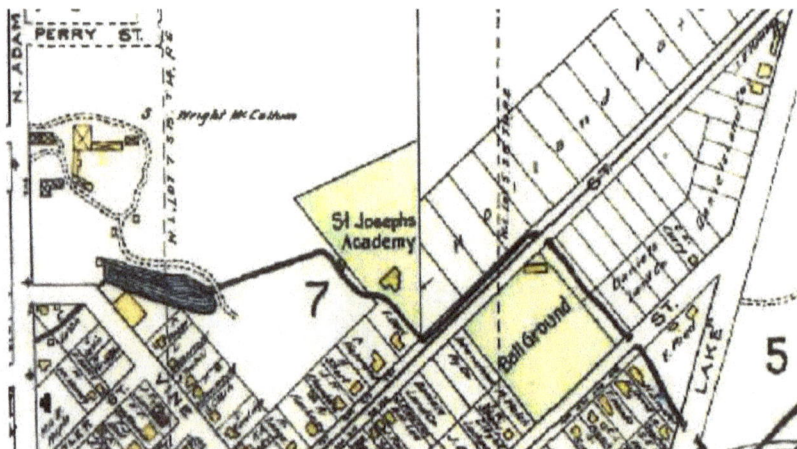

Lockport, New York 1908. St. Joseph's Academy and McCollum Farm.
Note the dark line of the tunnel that ran from the canal to the ice pond.

The spring on the property was believed to have healing properties. Following a European tradition of healing baths, the facility used methods developed by a German doctor, Dr. Sebastien's Kniepp. The therapy involved the application of water, hot and cold, at different pressures.

Through field work and discussions with Rich and Bree Woodbridge of the McCollum Farm, which borders the property, Ed Rice, another neighbor, and Sister Claire, Assistant Archivist of the Sisters of St. Mary of Namur, Kenmore, New York, we have a rough idea of where the spring was. The Niagara County Historian's Office also assisted with this research. Thank you to all.

Ed Rice, whose property includes some of the St. Joseph's land has faint outlines in the grass, during a dry summer, of the foundations of the old buildings. Both Ed Rice and Rich Woodbridge directed me to a small ravine with a flowing stream as the location of the spring. On the bank is a weathered built-in cement bench.

The area along Vine Street and part of Olcott Street are seasonally wet, which has made discovery of the spring difficult. Compounding this is an old tunnel to the McCollum Farm that is underground and reportedly runs from the canal under all the houses and streets. This tunnel was to fill the McCollum Farm ice pond, which still exists north of Vine Street. How functional the tunnel is after many years is not clear. The St. Joseph's spring water eventually ran into the ice pond.

It is believed that this tunnel still floods wooded areas on Vine Street and Olcott Street when the canal level is high. There are also reports of storm sewers that were directed to the area, much of which is a designated wet land.

Sleight's Mineral Baths
320 North Transit Street
Lockport, New York

This mineral bath was located in the cellar of 320 North Transit Street.

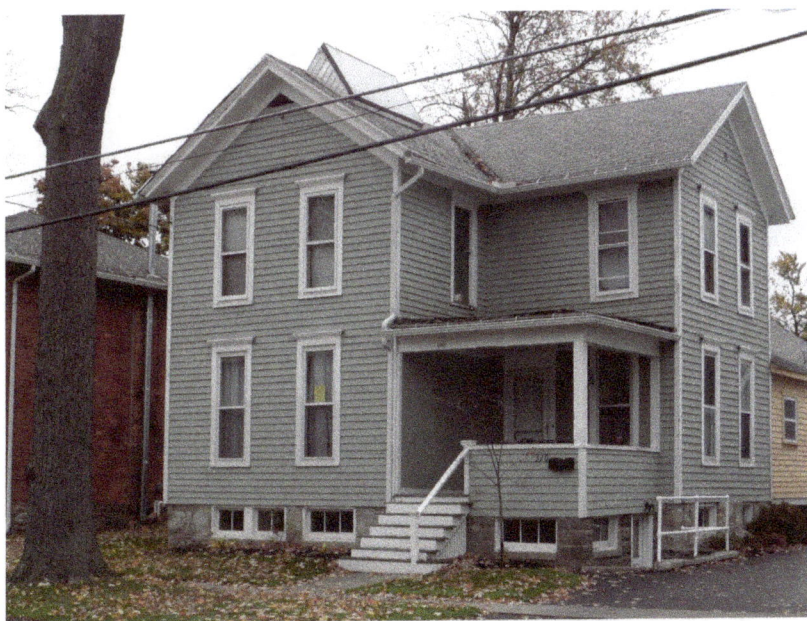

320 North Transit Street, Lockport, New York. Former location of Sleight's Mineral Baths. The external stairs to the basement was the patient entrance to the mineral baths.

Even eighty years later, it is possible to see that the bath would have looked luxurious. The basement had wall-to-wall ornate tile floor and dark wood paneling. There were radiators in each room and bright lighting. A special side entrance separated the facility from the house. It may have not been a European Spa, but it was the nearest that you could find in the North End of Lockport in the 1930s, the time of the Great Depression.

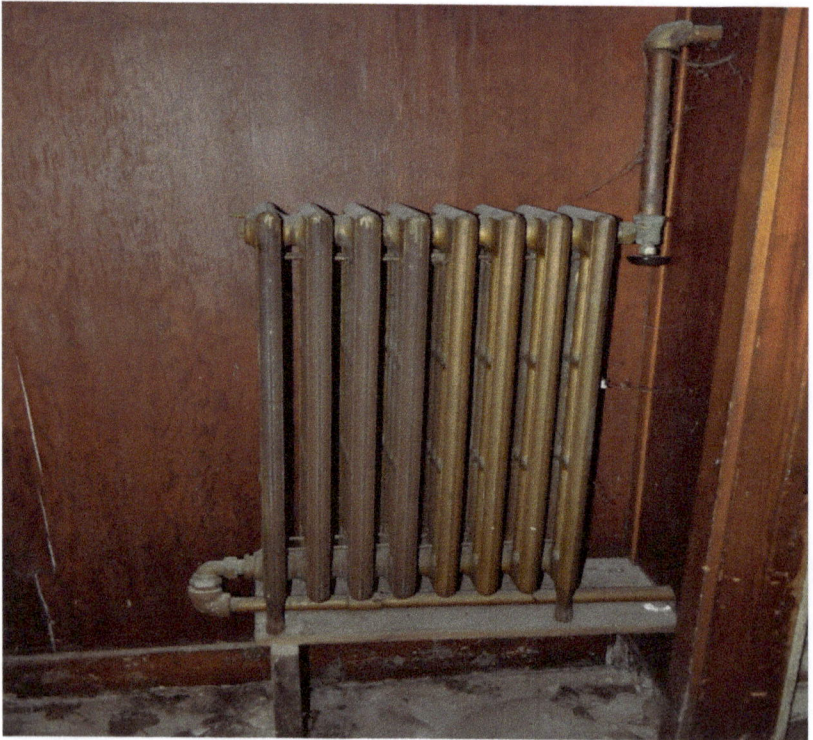

Wood paneling and radiators in the mineral baths.   *J. Boles 2016*

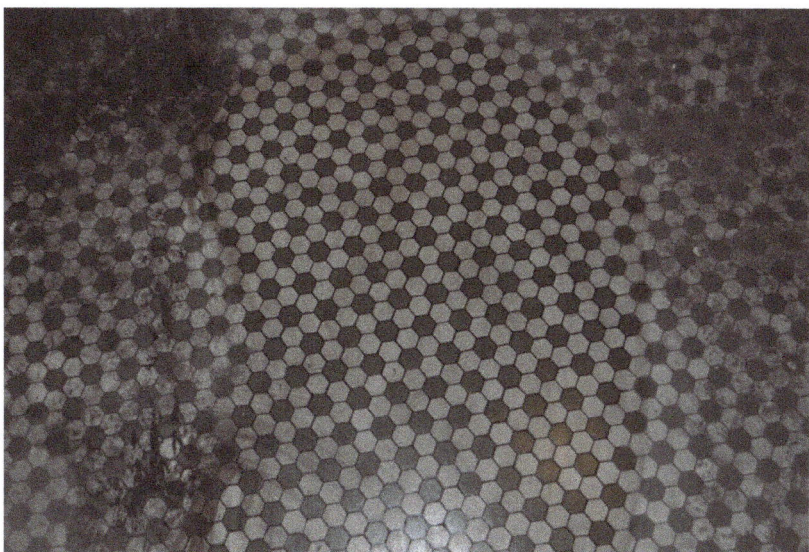

The basement has beautiful wall-to-wall ceramic tile from the former mineral bath.

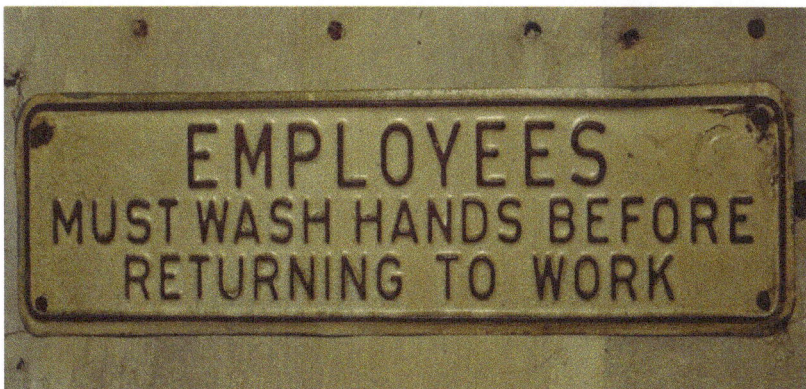

EMPLOYEES
MUST WASH HANDS BEFORE
RETURNING TO WORK

Sign in the bathroom of the mineral baths.

Jason and Jenna Walling, who purchased the old house in 2008 (built in 1860 by Michael Feeney) felt that, with the side entrance and the unusual cellar, the house must have a history. Jason, a "history buff," spent an afternoon at the Niagara County Historians Office. He commented, "they were very knowledgeable. Everyone pitched in, and within a few hours I had a complete history of the house and the Sleight Mineral Baths. What a great place."

The Sleight's Mineral Baths were opened in Lockport in 1934 by William Bickert, who purchased the house at 320 North Transit Street and installed the front entrance and outfitted the basement, turning it into a mineral bath. The equipment used was from a system sold out of Rochester, New York, by Earl V. Sleight. Mr. Sleight is believed to have derived his system from his previous employer, The John F. Class Bath Systems, Dayton Ohio. In the listings in the *Lockport Directory*, William Bickert is listed as a masseur and a magnetic healer. In theory, magnetic therapy works with the energy fields of the body to promote healing and may involve the use of magnets. The hands of the healer are used to assist in this process. The baths operated from 1934 to 1939. In 1940, Mr. Bickert moved on to another business, the Trade in Furniture Company, at 69 Market Street in Lockport.

With ads that compare the baths to the European Spas, the Sleights Mineral Baths had claims for a "True Natural means of preventing disease and also treating it." Further health claims included the improvement in all diseases, relief of neuritis (inflammation of the nervous system), arthritis, high blood pressure, sinus, and nervous disorders.

This bath was a typical hydropathy water cure of the time. It used water as a therapy to treat diseases or conditions. Usually mineral water—hot, tepid, and cold—was applied in baths, vapor baths, and under pressure as part of the treatments. Often other therapies and dietary recommendations were included.

MINERAL BATHS · 7

Sleight's Mineral Baths

Useful In ARTHRITIS, RHEUMATISM, COLDS, ASTHMA, NERVOUS CONDITIONS

HOURS 9 A. M.—8 P. M.

320 No. Transit St.   Phone 2152   Lockport, N. Y.

Lockport Directory 1937

Thank you to
- Christine L. Ridarsky, City Historian & Historical Svcs. Consultant, Rochester, New York
- Lockport Public Library Reference Librarians
- Niagara County Historian's Office
- Jason and Jenna Walling

Author's Notes

This book is one in a series to be published by Vanishing Past Press. The focus is on early local history, care and healing. A book titled *Tales from The Historic Springs, Niagara County, New York* will be out in October 2019. Future books under research, loosely titled, *The Poor Houses of Niagara County; Early Hospitals and Clinics, and Schools and Orphanages.* I may take a look at the large amount of research I have about Niagara County springs and produce a volume two about the history of our abundant springs. *The Keeley Gold Cures of New York State* is also in the works and it takes a broader look at these 1890's addiction cures that I first wrote about in "The Gold Cure Institutes of Niagara Falls, New York" in 2013.

Readers are encouraged to contact me with further information or questions at jamesboles47@gmail.com.

Other Titles by Jim Boles

Dr Skinners Remarkable School for "Colored Deaf and Dumb, and Blind Children, James M. Boles and Michael Boston

When There Were Poorhouses

The Gold Cure Institutes of Niagara Falls, NY

They Did No Harm-Alternative Medicine in Niagara Falls, NY

Abandoned History, Lockport New York 2017

Ivan the Invacar Series: children's books-disability related

Contributed:

On The Edge of Town: Almshouses of Western New York -Publisher

No Offense Intended: A Directory of Historical Disability Terms -Editor

Abandoned Asylums of New England: A Photographic Journey by John Gray -Publisher

Buffalo State Hospital: A History of the Institution in Light and Shadow, published by the Museum of disABILITY History, Buffalo New York -Contributor

J.N Adams Memorial Hospital-Her Inside Voice by Char Szabo-Perricelli, published by the Museum of disABILITY History, Buffalo New York -Publisher, editor

Buffalo State Psychiatric Hospital: An Inside Report from the 1950s, by Patricia Kautz, published by the Museum of disABILITY History -Contributor

Path to the Institution: The New York State Asylum for Idiots by Thomas E. Stearns -Executive Editor

Beautiful Children: The story of the Elm Hill School and home for Feebleminded Children and Youth by Diana M. Katovitch -Editor

Of Grave Importance: The Restoration of Institutional Cemeteries by David Mack-Hardiman

www.ingramcontent.com/pod-product-compliance
Lightning Source LLC
Chambersburg PA
CBHW051300020426
42333CB00026B/3288